Dedication

To the parents who once cradled their child and, without words, made a promise to protect, to nourish, and to give what was needed—especially sleep. In those first months, you knew: Sleep was sacred. It was growth. It was love. But life crept in. Bedtimes stretched. And the quiet wisdom of Sleep Wellness gave way to the glow of screens and late-night habits. May this guide serve as a return, a remembrance, and a gift for you and your child to allow sleep to be love again.

To all the parents who think, *"Why not let the kids stay up late and have some grown-up fun? What harm can it do?"* may this Guide remind you that, like most grown-up fun, there are consequences that are all the more detrimental to maturing brains.

And to all the adults in the household who think they were born '*night owls,*' believe they *do their best work when everyone else is asleep*, and relish catching their '*second wind*' for the '*me-time*' they deserve, may this Guide be your '**wake-up call**' to reclaim your birthright to Sleep Wellness for yourself and all your loved ones!

Embracing Sleep Wellness; A Family Guide To Transforming Sleep Resistance Into A Nurturing Ritual

Copyright ©2025
ISBN: 979-8-9888471-5-1

All rights reserved.
No part of this book may be reproduced or used in any manner without express written permission from the copyright holders.
Publisher: Sleep To Live Well Foundation
City, State: San Jose, California, United States
Contact info: info@sleeptolivewell.org

PARENTS GUIDE TO SLEEP WELLNESS **SLEEP TO LIVE WELL FOUNDATION**

Using This Guide
Designed to Support the Household As Needs Arise and Evolve

Part 1: Introduction — Pages 3 - 11

Start here to meet Sleep-Wellness Advisor Roger Washington, MD, and be reminded of how essential sleep is to the health and well-being of all creatures, especially humans. Find here the easy to read list of the primary benefits of sufficient sleep, the dangers of insufficient sleep for the children in your life, and the ways Sleep Wellness practices support all members of your household.

Part 2: The Importance of Sleep Wellness — Pages 12 - 14

Come to this section to be reminded that Sleep Wellness is FREE. So, no matter your circumstances, you can prioritize quality sleep and learn how to make sure your child receives their complete sleep quota to stay healthy and happy.

Part 3: Unlearn Bad Habits You Were Taught As A Child — Pages 15 - 24

In this section, you may be surprised to discover how your bedtime habits as an adult were formed in childhood! Recognizing your sleep dysfunctions is an important step toward making Sleep Wellness practices successful in your home, especially for young children. You will learn how to teach what you may not have learned in a more natural way, making it easier for your child to embrace bedtime and wake up rejuvenated and eager to take on the day.

Part 4: Good Sleep Wellness Habits and How To Teach Them — Pages 25 - 40

This is the section where all the good Sleep Wellness practices are outlined, and you are given ways to implement them so you can feel confident in knowing what your child's sleep needs are and in helping them recognize those needs as well. This is also the part where you will learn how to incorporate emotional nurturing into bedtime routines, which will strengthen your bond with your child throughout their journey into adulthood.

Part 5: Set A Good Example: Support for Adults in the Household — Pages 41 - 54

Come to this section to receive the compassion you deserve. As adults, many of us have inherited sleep struggles shaped by cultural myths, life demands, and childhood patterns we adopted with the understanding of a child, accepting them as normal—without realizing the cost. This section offers you grace—not guilt—and practical tools to begin healing your own sleep issues while protecting your children from the same generational burdens. You will find science-backed insights, empowering reminders, and emotional encouragement to reclaim Sleep Wellness as an act of love—for yourself and for those you care for.

FAQs, Glossary, Children's Book, Invitation to Support Sleep To Live Well — Pages 55 - 64

Part 1

PARENTS GUIDE TO SLEEP WELLNESS — **SLEEP TO LIVE WELL FOUNDATION**

INTRODUCTION

Meet Sleep-Wellness Advisor Roger Washington, MD (Page 4)

Regardless of your circumstances YOU CAN prioritize Sleep Wellness with other parental responsibilities. (Page 5)

Benefits of Sufficient Sleep for Children (Page 6-7)

Dangers of Insufficient Sleep for Children (Page 8-9)

How Sleep Wellness Benefits the Entire Family (Page 10-11)

INTRODUCTION

Hello, I'm Roger Washington, MD, aka "Doctor Bedtime"

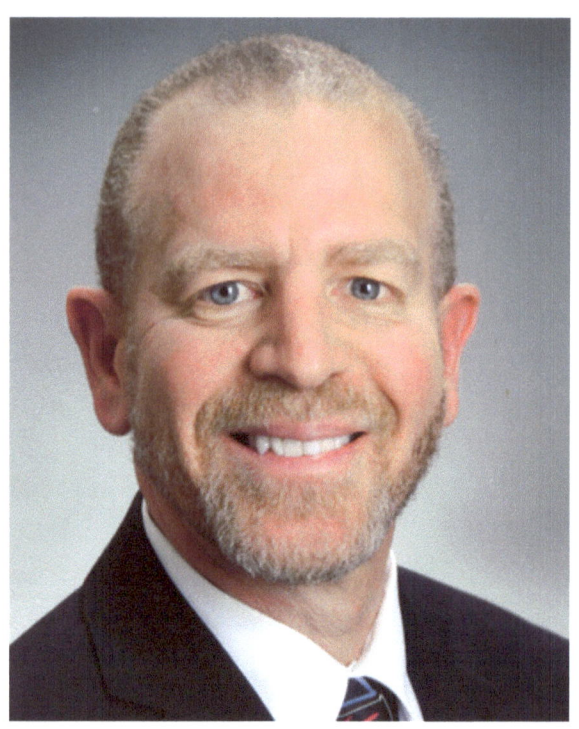

I established the Sleep To Live Well Foundation to sound the alarm that ignoring Sleep Wellness has dire health consequences—especially for our children, who need sleep's growth and repair superpower the most. Our educational resources encourage children and their caregivers—parents and physicians—to entrain and model Sleep Wellness for our children.

Thank you for joining us!

As a family physician for more than 30 years, I emphasized the importance of sleep in discussions with patients in my primary care practice. In addition to my outstanding training at Stanford University Medical School, I developed a holistic approach and made Sleep Wellness a primary screening tool and treatment in my medicine bag.

The **lack of sufficient sleep (LOSS)** became a crucial factor in diagnosing illnesses and led to my discovery that insufficient sleep is the root cause of what we call disease.

I researched the consistent link between LOSS and sickness and documented how and when LOSS inevitably sparks illness and disease.

I observed how LOSS not only weakened my patients' immune systems, but also reflexively triggered inflammatory diseases of all severities, such as heart attacks, strokes, migraines, seizures, multiple sclerosis, asthma, eczema, psoriasis, gout and stones. And it reflexively triggered insulin resistance, weight gain, and diabetes.

Regardless of your circumstances - <u>YOU CAN prioritize Sleep Wellness</u> with other responsibilities.

Sleep is an essential physiologic need for children, just as important as food and water. However, many parents may struggle with maintaining Sleep Wellness in their households, even though they have the financial means to provide for their child's basic and essential needs. Conversely, some parents may face financial difficulties and other hardships, but can still instill healthy sleep habits in their children.

This Sleep-Wellness Guide aims to help you prioritize Sleep Wellness and practice it with the same vigor, enthusiasm, love, and sense of duty you devote to meeting your children's other essential needs.

Sleep is essential for the growth and repair of the body and mind. It is not *rest*. It is far more important and instrumental.

Deep sleep is crucial for enabling the body to repair and replace cells as they degrade. It stimulates physical growth and mental and emotional balance. Sufficient sleep builds resilience to stress and strength to rebound from trauma.

Sleep Wellness allows us to sustain life and promotes a sense of well-being. It is the ultimate Preventive Medicine. Sleep Wellness improves the quality of your child's life.

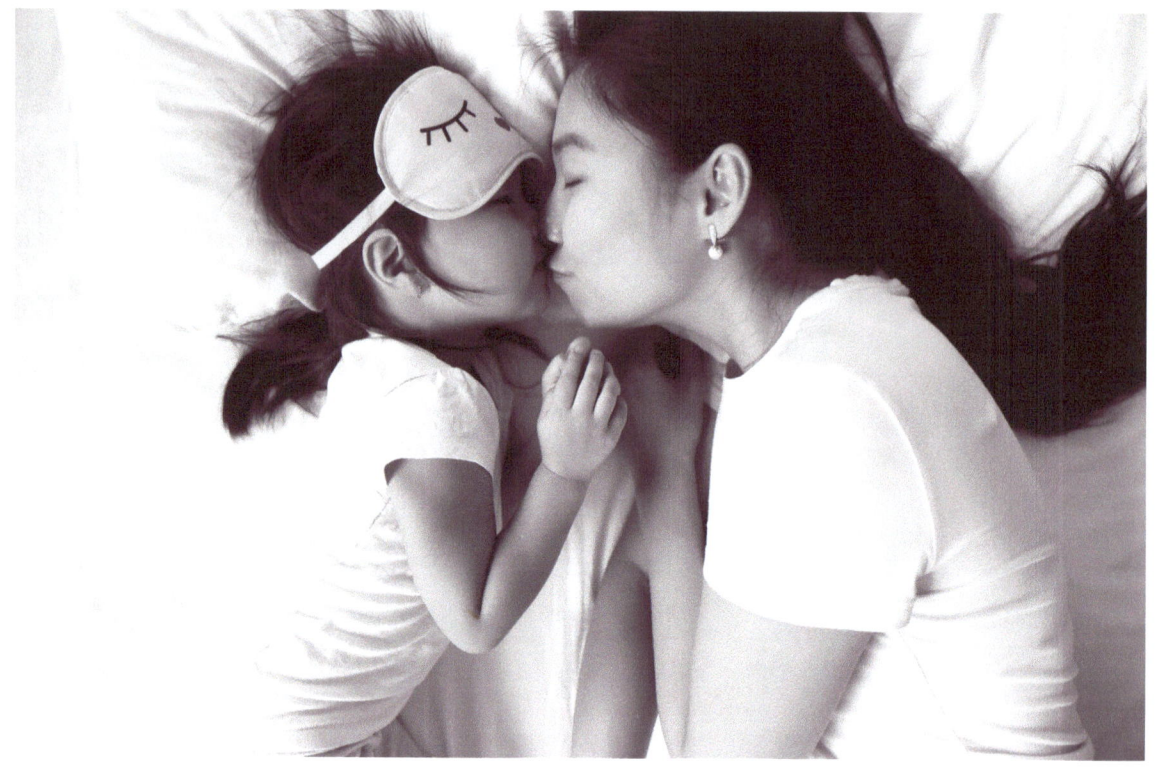

You can enhance a child's future without spending a penny. Give them good bedtime habits and Sleep Wellness practices that will last a lifetime!

Children who get the sleep they need are more likely to:

ENJOY LIFE
- Wake up happier, less grumpy
- Feel energized/eager to face the day
- Make better decisions about wellbeing
- Be joyful and share happiness
- Thrive mentally and emotionally

BE HEALTHY
- Grow to their full potential height
- Have a good appetite
- Resist illnesses and heal faster
- Be resilient and cope with adversity
- Have more confidence/be less fearful

LEARN BETTER
- Perform easier and better at school
- Memorize lessons and recall advice
- Accept disappointment and move on

BEHAVE BETTER
- Not feel bored or act impulsively
- Not be reckless
- Not pout, sulk, or remain angry
- Not disobey the rules and act out

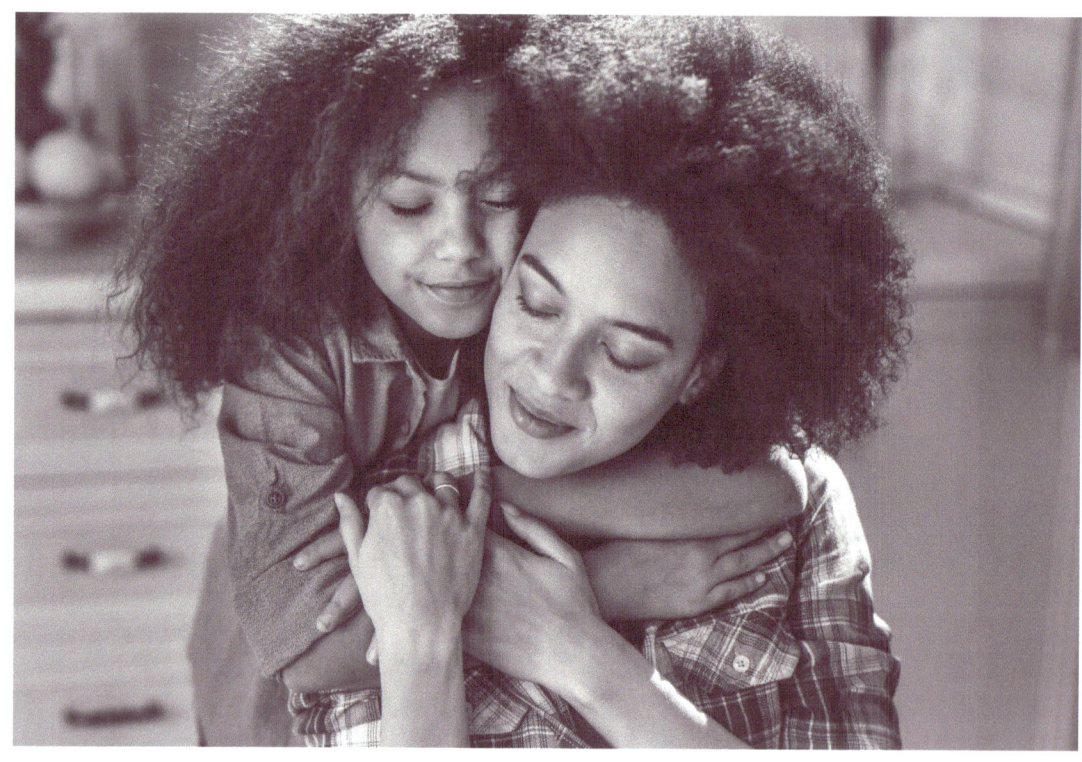

Sleep Wellness practices benefit parents and the entire family by allowing you to sustain life, promote a sense of well-being, and improve the quality of your child's life. <u>Sleep Wellness IS Preventive Medicine.</u>

Sleep Wellness benefits the entire family. Sufficient sleep and bedtime rituals can:

CREATE A PEACEFUL HOME
- Less resistance to bedtime schedules and rules
- A calm household helps the family face challenges outside the home

SAVE MONEY
- Fewer sick days, less time missed at work and school
- Faster recovery from illnesses, which means less money on doctor visits and medicine

CREATE PROUD PARENTS
- Seeing children grow to their full potential – physically, mentally, and emotionally – is rewarding
- The joy of seeing children sleep deeply and soundly builds confidence in parenting skills

BUILD A STRONGER FAMILY
- Foster stability and a sense of security and belonging
- Strengthen family bonds
- Transfer Sleep Wellness practices to children for a lifetime of benefits

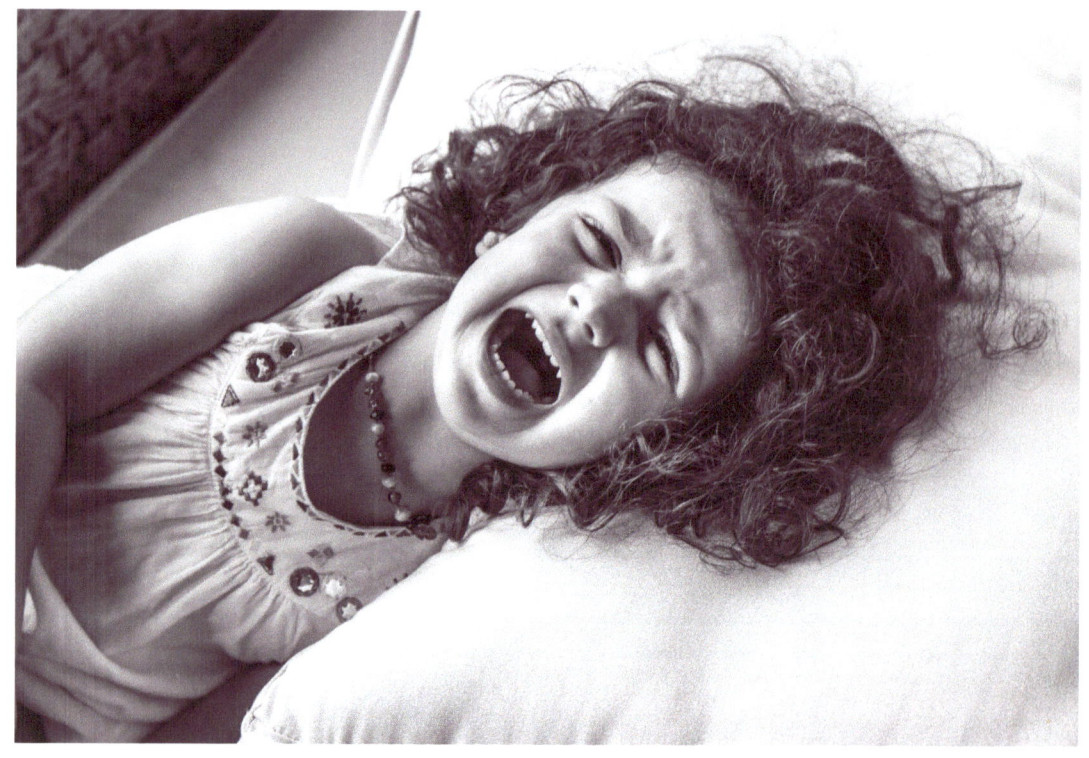

Insufficient sleep is costly to everyone.
It impacts children, families, and society as a whole.

Insufficient sleep is dangerous. Without the right amount of sleep, children are more likely to:

BEHAVE BADLY
- Show aggression toward others
- Engage in risky behaviors
- Break rules and not respect authority
- Experiment with alcohol and drugs

DIFFICULTY LEARNING
- Have learning problems
- Make poor decisions
- Lack problem-solving skills

BE LESS HEALTHY
- Be more susceptible to illnesses
- Heal slower
- Suffer from stunted growth—physically, mentally, and emotionally
- Lack a hearty appetite
- Crave junk food

STRUGGLE MORE
- Be mentally and emotionally unstable
- Often be irritable, frustrated, and bored
- Have more bouts of depression
- Lack self-esteem and self-confidence

Part 2

THE IMPORTANCE OF SLEEP WELLNESS

1: Sleep Wellness is FREE. (Page 13)

2: PRIORITIZE Sleep Wellness. (Page 13)

3: Learn to allow your child their complete sleep quota. (Page 14)

1: Sleep Wellness is FREE

All creatures on Earth are born with the innate capacity to reconnect to the source of all life--for growth, restoration, repair, and healing-- through sleep. We humans are the only beings who can fool ourselves into thinking we can take a pass on sleep without consequences

Sleep is your birthright to energy, waiting to be inherited.

The Sleep Wellness practices in this guide will help you sustain your child's innate need for connection to life-giving sleep. It is one of the greatest gifts you can give as a parent, and unlike food and water in our society, sleep is still FREE. Teaching your child to be aware, appreciative, and empowered by sleep is an invaluable gift that lays the foundation for a life well-lived.

2: PRIORITIZE Sleep Wellness

Parental instincts are to provide for children's needs. We feed, clothe, and protect them from harm, provide for their learning, enrich their life experiences, and make them happy so they can grow healthy, strong, and capable of caring for themselves. We shower them with expressions of our love to the extent we can. We would never *intentionally* give them less food and water than they require or underdress them for cold weather.

Children need their full quota of sleep to maintain their mental, physical, and emotional health and balance.

Even if you prioritize sleep among your other parental responsibilities, it is difficult to recognize when children are getting the full quota, especially as they age. But as you learn the principles of Sleep Wellness, you will be empowered to recognize the amount of sleep your child needs from day to day to be healthy and happy.

3: Learn to allow your child their complete sleep quota.

Sleep Wellness begins with learning your child's cues to gauge their sleep needs. You can do this while creating a physically and emotionally safe, secure, and comfortable environment conducive to sleeping sufficiently.

*"Traditionally, for reasons that still baffle me, childcare professionals do not consider a child's complete **sleep quota** as one of the most basic physiological needs," said Dr. Washington.*

"Medical school does not train doctors to ensure sleep sufficiency and satiation. Eventually, the change will happen, but only when parents demand it," he added.

It is not your fault that you have not learned to maintain sleep sufficiency throughout your child's growth cycles and development. Sleep Wellness is not ingrained in most parents.

But you have transferrable practices: Based on your observations of their behaviors and your best judgment, you know what your child's behavior is when they are hungry, have not eaten enough, are too cold, or are too warm. However, you are less likely to observe whether they sleep sufficiently after infancy.

This guide will teach you to observe your children closely for the signs that they need sleep or the vital signs they have slept insufficiently, which is critical to getting their sleep needs met – from one sleep and wake cycle to the next. You can learn to ensure your child gets their full sleep quota as they grow and mature.

Part 3

UNLEARN BAD HABITS YOU WERE TAUGHT AS A CHILD

4: Don't make bedtime and sleep a punishment. (Page 16-17)

5: Learn to make bedtime safe, sacred. and loving. (Page 18-19)

6: Don't indulge children's desire to stay up past bedtime. (Page 20-21)

7: Younger children REQUIRE a different sleep schedule than older siblings. (Page 22-23)

8: Lead by example OR pay the price. (Page 24)

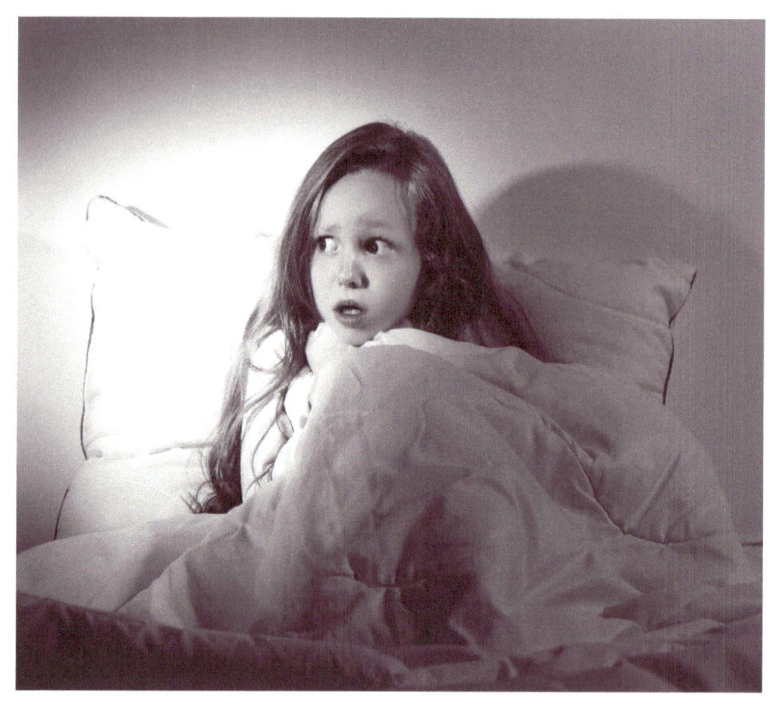

There are habits you learned that sabotage Sleep Wellness in your household. <u>Don't make bedtime or sleep a punishment.</u>

4: It is never too late to unlearn bad habits and practice good Sleep Wellness habits.

Many adults learned the bad habit of using bedtime as a punishment because that's how they were treated as a child.
Does this sound familiar to you?

> *If you don't behave, you'll have to go to bed!*
> *You didn't stop when I told you, so go to bed!*
> *You're being a bad (boy, girl). Now go to bed!*
> *You are getting on my nerves. Go to bed!*

No doubt, parents of your generation and those before yours experienced negative bedtime associations like the ones above as children--or worse. No wonder you stay up as long as possible to feel a sense of freedom and catch that *second wind,* which then does you in the following day by affecting your mood and diminishing your mental sharpness.

Parents: Do not pass this bad habit of punishing your child with bedtime on to your children.

Using bedtime as punishment creates the worst association for Sleep Wellness, which can wound them for life. Find other ways to discipline your child—time out in the corner, less time on their screens, on the phone, or in after-school activities—please do not mar the bedtime and sleep experience.

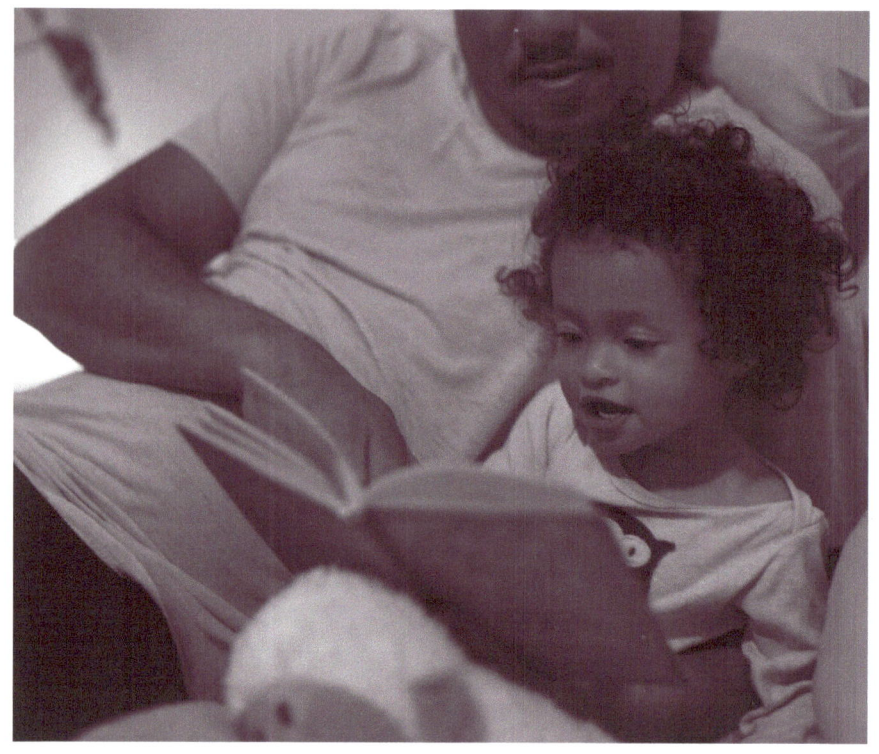

<u>Making bedtime safe, sacred, and loving can have long-lasting rewards.</u> After all, this is where children must go to grow bigger and stronger, heal if they are sick, and ease their minds and emotions if they are troubled.

5: Make bedtime safe, sacred, and loving.

Another sabotaging sleep habit parents may unintentionally allow in their household is ignoring the sacredness of bedtime and not ensuring the child's sleeping space feels safe.

Here's the advice you need to turn this around:

- All creatures need and seek a safe place to sleep at night. When you are mindful of providing one for your child, you enhance your covenant as a parent.

- A child's sleep space does not have to be elaborate; what passes for comfort differs from one family to another. But the sleep space you create for your child should feel special and as safe as you can possibly make it.

- Teaching your child to covet, value, and protect their safe space for sleeping, no matter how grand or meager, is a lesson that will stay with them and support them throughout their lives.

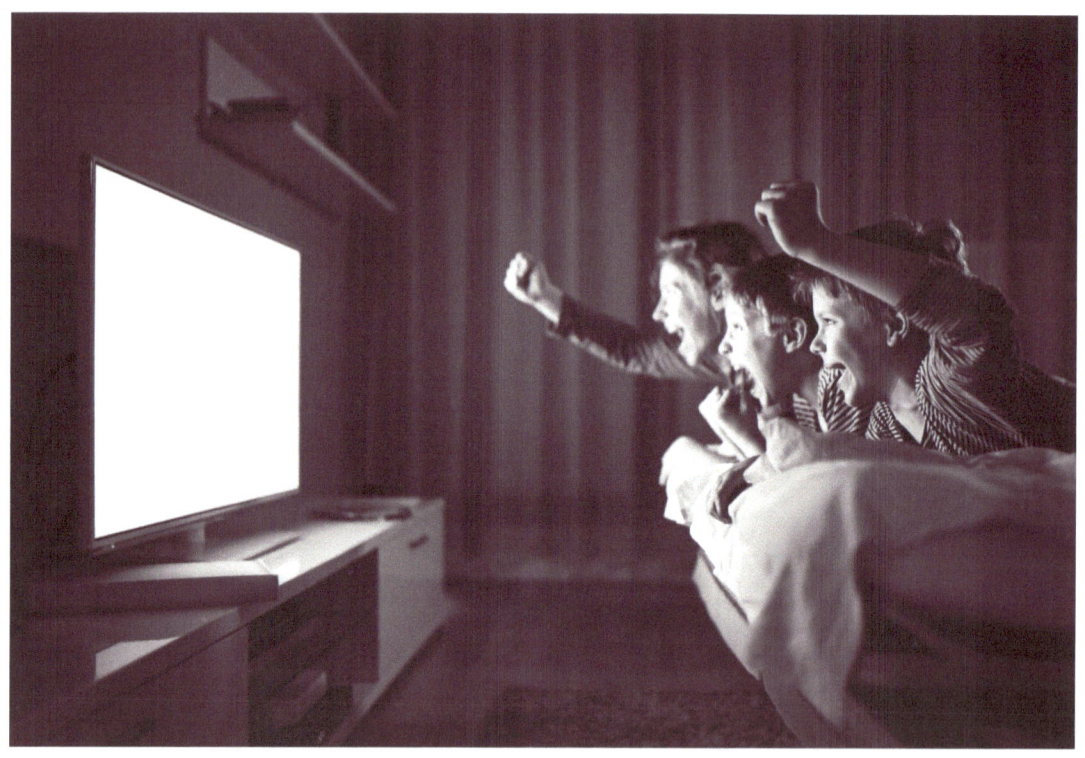

<u>Allowing children to stay up late is a bad habit.</u> No matter how much they enjoy it, you are compromising their need for sleep and, as a result, their health.

6: Don't indulge children's desire to stay up past their bedtime.

Many parents are guilty of this bad habit, but it is not your fault! Sleep Wellness can help you break the cycle if you experienced this BAD habit as a child.

Some parents feel the risk of staying up late is small, and the pleasure children experience is a worthwhile part of their cultural experience. They may think introducing them to staying up past their known bedtime at a young age on weekends or special occasions is okay, but it should not be encouraged or given as a treat.

However, in children of all ages, staying up late decreases the amount of deep and REM sleep, the sleep stages responsible for physical and mental growth. Staying up late is especially hazardous for newborns because it greatly increases the risk of crib death or Sudden Infant Death Syndrome (SIDs).

A study showed that infants whose sleep schedule has been delayed by just 2 hours stop breathing more often and are more difficult to awaken.

"I am baffled by why more pediatricians and family physicians are not alarmed by the risks associated with delayed and erratic sleeping patterns," said Dr. Washington. "In every case, spending less time in crucial sleep cycles damages growing children."

Allowing your child to stay up late on weekends and during family vacations is a bad habit because it instills in children's minds that their early bedtime is just for school. They are not learning to associate sleep with all its superpowers, including growing, healing, and building resilience, which are vital powers at a young age.

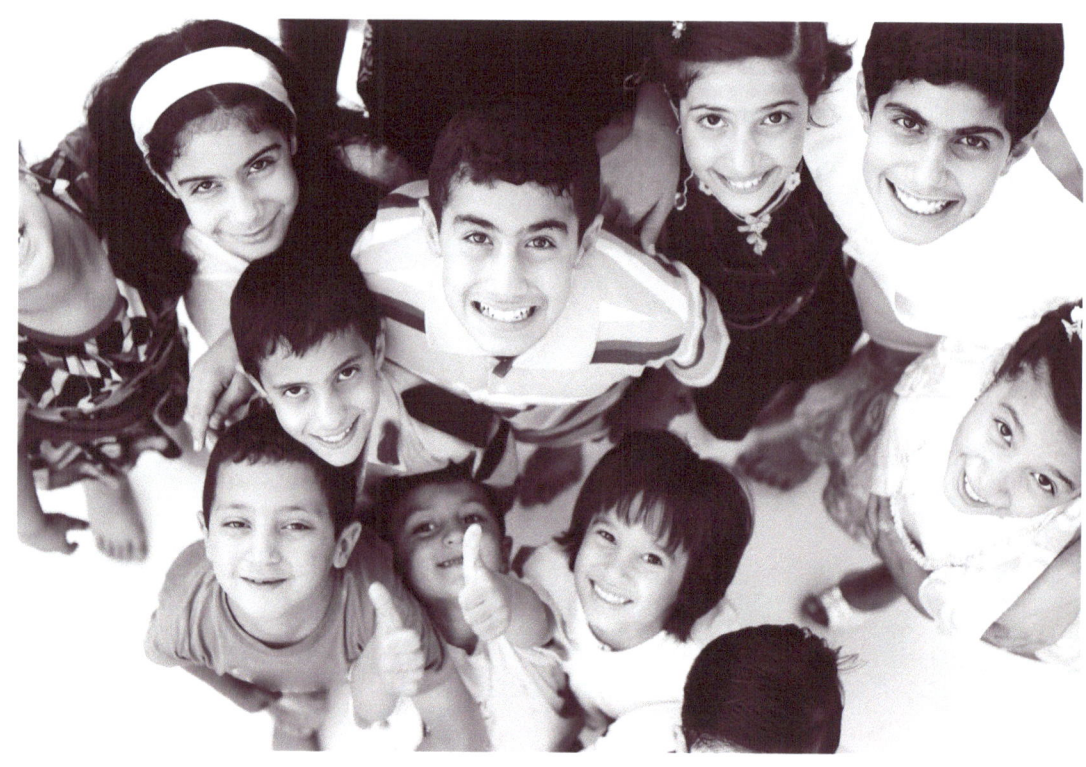

A child's notion of what is "fair" is immature. Having different bedtimes for different ages is a teaching opportunity. Communicate that your rules may differ, but your love is the same.

7: Younger children REQUIRE a different sleep schedule than older siblings.

They may not realize it now, but the healthy bedtime routine you are instilling is an example of your love and sense of duty.

Granted, if it has not been a habit in the household from the start, it may be challenging to enforce. However, you can accomplish a varied sleep time by using consistency and tools, such as night masks and headphones, and rewarding compliance.

Here are tips to stagger bedtimes:

- Make bedtime rituals special for each age group. Draw your children into their bedtime schedule with engaging activities just for them.

- Activities like reading and coloring can put younger children on their special track to sleep.

- If children of different ages share a sleeping area, the younger ones can wear eye masks to shield them from light, age-appropriate ear protection to decrease the noise, and the older ones can learn to respect quiet time.

- In a household with young children, turning screens off and lights out at a reasonable time for older siblings AND adults promotes Sleep Wellness for the entire family.

8: Lead by example OR pay the price.

Parents: Lead by example. It is one thing to stay up late for one's job or household tasks that cannot wait until morning, but staying up late for recreational activities sets a bad example for your family.

You squander the family's effectiveness and enthusiasm when you are too tired to be fully present in the morning. Your drowsiness compromises your ability to be attentive, anticipate their needs, and lead them by enthusiastic example.

Your children will notice and eventually mimic you. By showing your family how to reap the benefits of sleep, you set a good example.

ASK YOURSELF...

- *"Do I want to teach my child that being tired in the morning is normal?*

- *"Do I want to model drudgery or model gratitude and cheerfulness?"*

Perhaps you learned poor sleep habits from your parents. Regardless, now that you are more aware of their ill effects, your children will appreciate the difference when you awake feeling present and capable.

Sleep Wellness can help you break the cycle if you experienced bad sleep habits as a child around your parents.

Part 4

GOOD HABITS AND HOW TO TEACH THEM

9: Recognize your child's sleep cues. (Page 26-27)

10: Teach your child to know their sleep cues and how to use them. (Page 28-29)

11: Begin the bedtime rituals for winding down when sleep cues appear. (Page 30)

12: Be flexible to accommodate your child's need to sleep earlier than usual. (Page 31)

13: Set the intention to make bedtime an emotional check-in with your child. (Page 32-33)

14: Reframe your child's frustrations before sleep to encourage emotional health and maturity. (Page 34-35)

15: Allow your child to sleep undisturbed until they awake naturally, as often as possible. (Page 36-37)

16: Call attention to how well your child feels when they have a good nap or night's sleep and awaken refreshed. (Page 38-39)

17: Provide a secure haven where your child can tap into the wonders and magic of sleep. (Page 40)

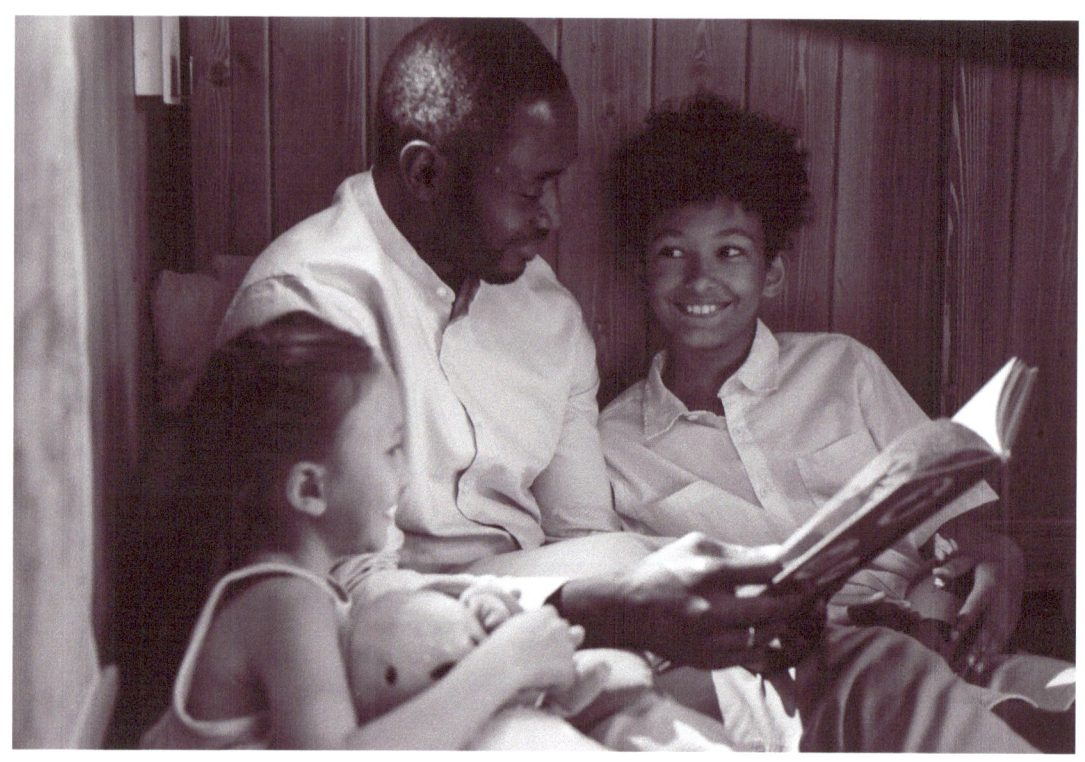

You are very lucky if you've already learned Sleep Wellness habits. <u>Adopting new behaviors is possible at any age, even if you didn't experience great bedtime habits as a child.</u>

9: Recognize your child's sleep cues.

It started when you were a baby. As a newborn, your parents paid attention to every little thing, especially if you were the first. By observing you closely, they learn your language for hunger, discomfort, pain, and tiredness.

Likewise, observe when your child is getting sleepy and the behavior pattern that follows before going to sleep. This is an essential early habit for establishing Sleep Wellness in your family.

Children's *sleep cues* and sleeping patterns remain the same over long periods.

Knowing their *sleep language* alerts you to their *sleep window opening*, which allows you to be proactive before the window of opportunity to sleep well closes.

> **This guide explains the sleep window, coined the *Washington Sleep Wellness Window*, and the hazardous consequences for children and adults who stay awake after their sleep window closes.**

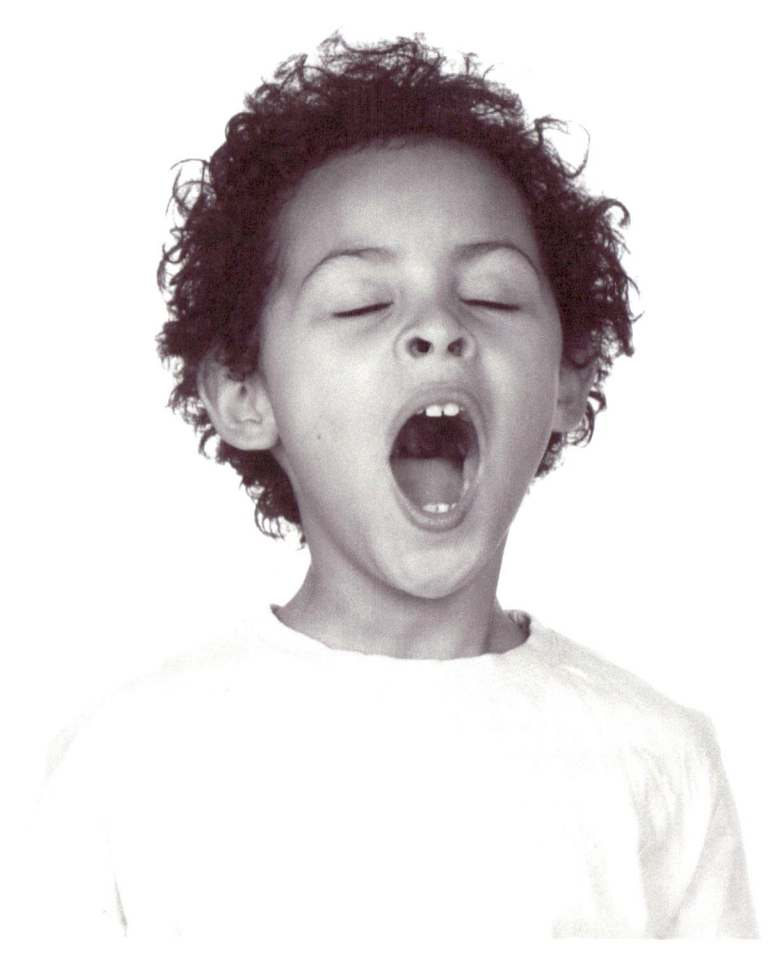

<u>Teach your child to interpret their feelings</u> of drowsiness, yawning, scratching their heads, and rubbing their eyes as signs that their bodies need sleep.

10: Teach your child to identify their sleep cues and know how to use them.

Mirroring sleep cues to your children encourages self-awareness and, eventually, self-care.

Start by observing your child yawning, head-scratching, stretching, and eye-rubbing, and then subtly let your body reflect their movements. If they yawn, then you yawn. If they stretch, then you do the same.

Mirroring your child's facial expressions and body positions instantly communicates empathy and signals that you understand their feelings and will consider them. Then, you can point out the cues you observe, increasing their awareness of them and how they affect their feelings. Let them know it is time for bed because their body is ready for sleep.

Young children may not always be aware of cues that indicate their basic needs, such as hunger, urination, or defecation, until someone points them out.

As they become more familiar with these contrasting sensations, they can use them as effective tools to self-regulate their behavior. They can embrace their natural urge to sleep, like learning to use the potty. After sleeping, point out how they feel "better", more energetic and happy.

> **You are teaching your child to interpret their feelings of drowsiness and their actions of yawning, scratching their heads, and rubbing their eyes as signs that their bodies need sleep. It's a lesson of self-awareness that will serve them well throughout their entire life.**

11: Begin the bedtime rituals for winding down when sleep cues appear.

Consistently initiating a power-down period with winding-down rituals, as sleep cues begin, gives children structure and a sense of security before bedtime, as they know what to expect.

A wind-down before bedtime is important because it helps AVOID:

- **Putting the child to bed late**
- **Missing their window of opportunity to sleep well**
- **Getting overly Tired and Cranky - *"TRANKY"***
- **Becoming vulnerable to illness.**

Vacillating about when to prepare for sleep and not being attentive to the cues conveys to your child that you do not feel sleep rules are essential.

Suppose your child gets away with staying up one night or two and enjoys. In that case, they will start to look forward to being up past their bedtime and behave as anyone does when given intermittent positive reinforcement—you want more.

When your child stays up past their natural sleep wellness window, they are likely get a burst of energy known as "the second wind." It feels exciting, like a treat, and that rush creates an addictive craving. When bedtime becomes negotiable, kids start to chase that feeling. Staying consistent helps children, and adults, fall asleep more easily and keeps natural rhythms on track.

12: Be flexible to accommodate your child's need to sleep earlier than usual.

The amount of sleep your child needs for additional growth and repair is prompted by their increased physical and mental activity. For example, swimming and running usually cause children to sleep more than their usual quota.

Preparing for an *earlier* sleep time in those situations is a strategic way to provide more sleep when required.

Even an increase in the day's mental activities can cause the Washington Sleep Wellness Window to open early.

Just as you would anticipate your child will be thirstier and require more water after playing in the sun, you should prepare for their increased need for sleep after a big activity day.

The rule of going to sleep at the same time each night is a sleep-hygiene principle meant to improve insomnia, whereas Sleep Wellness aims to bring you into balance with your sleep needs. You should not always apply this overly simplistic rule to your growing child, who may need to get into bed earlier and go to sleep earlier for more sleep, so be flexible with starting their bedtime preparation sooner.

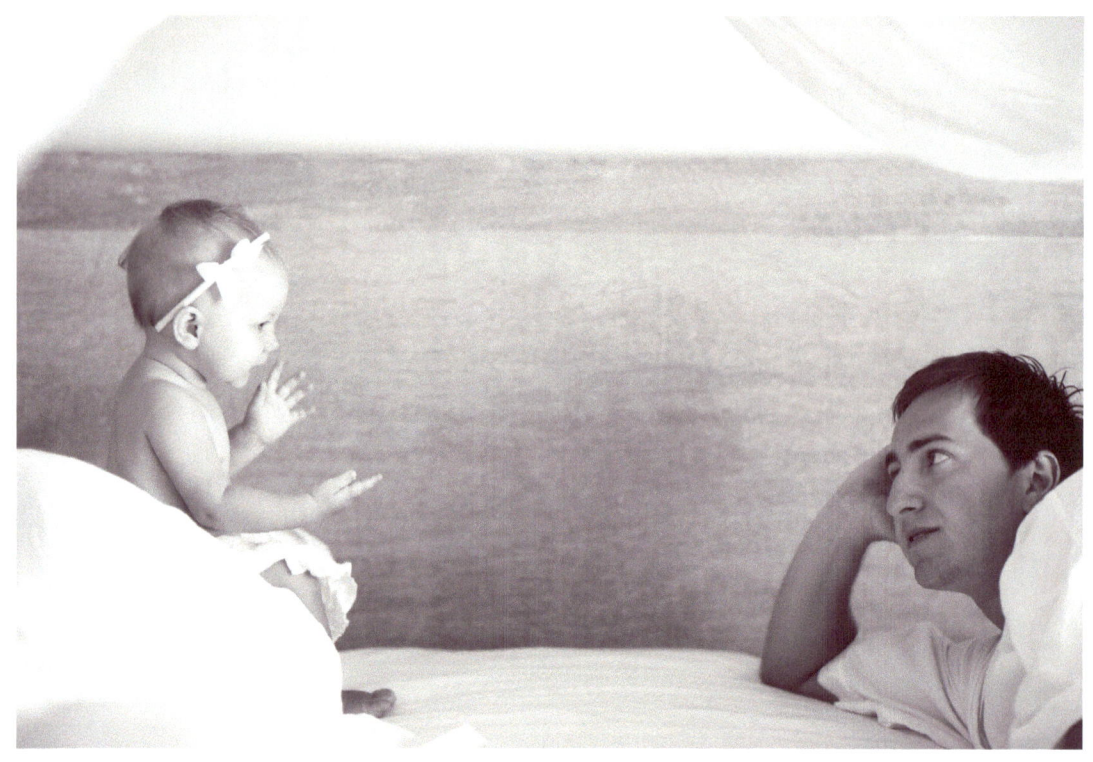

Create a habit of reading a bedtime story AND listening to your child before sleeping. This emotional check-in eases their burdens and supports growth and development on multiple levels.

13: Set the intention to make bedtime an emotional check-in with your child.

> **The benefits of an emotional check-in create a positive chain reaction.**

Bedtime stories and encouragement before bed help their natural attitude of gratitude and belonging emerge.

Gratitude displaces feelings of frustration, irritability, and a sense of lack.

Feeling more hopeful, children let go of churning emotional problems and mental worries that lead to nightmares and restless sleep.

With fewer emotional burdens, more precious time is allotted to fun dreams, learning, rejuvenating repairs and physical and emotional growth from quality sleep.

Rejuvenation empowers your child to wake up feeling refreshed, optimistic, content, and happy, which builds their resilience to overcome the challenges they face in life.

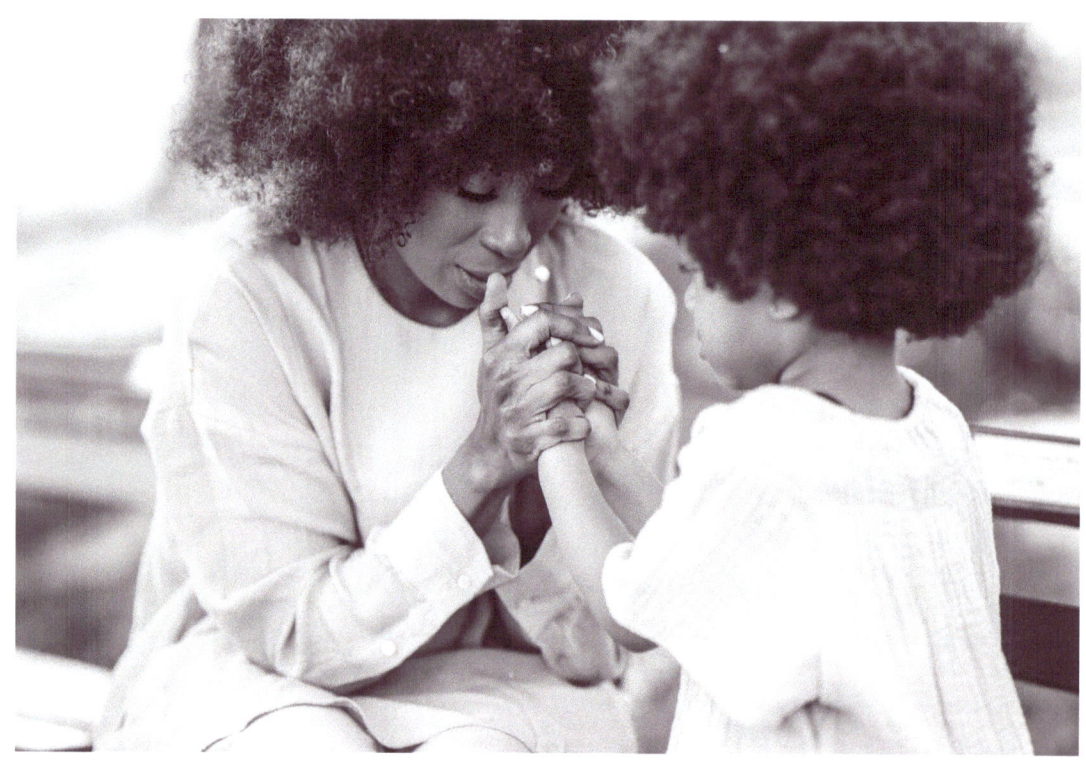

The practice of gratitude positively reframes your child's experiences. This is as soothing - like a prayer before bedtime. It can transform distress into a more mature and constructive interpretation. This realigns thoughts and calms stress.

14: Reframe frustrations before sleep to encourage emotional health and maturity.

A before-bed meeting with your child tends to help rectify a tendency to misinterpret the day's frustrating occurrences and circumstances. Instead of the child falling asleep without addressing their perceived problems and immature inferences, an adult perspective can realign their thinking and allay their concerns.

A child deciding, for example, that *Nana doesn't love me anymore* because of a forgotten birthday or *my best friend hates me* because of some perceived slight or insult, are not the kind of feelings or ideas to go to sleep with or incorporate more vividly into their worldview.

Reframing their perspective with a more mature, helpful interpretation is essential to healthy emotional growth. In this instance, you can help your child learn to forgive and accept that Gramma or their best friend made a mistake, but their mistakes do not entirely define them. This will enable your child to release the perceived hurt before bed, which can reaffirm connection and affection for their loved ones.

> **In some families, it is called praying before sleep and usually involves applying *principles of gratitude*, dispensing forgiveness, feeling forgiven, and the encouragement that they belong and are loved.**

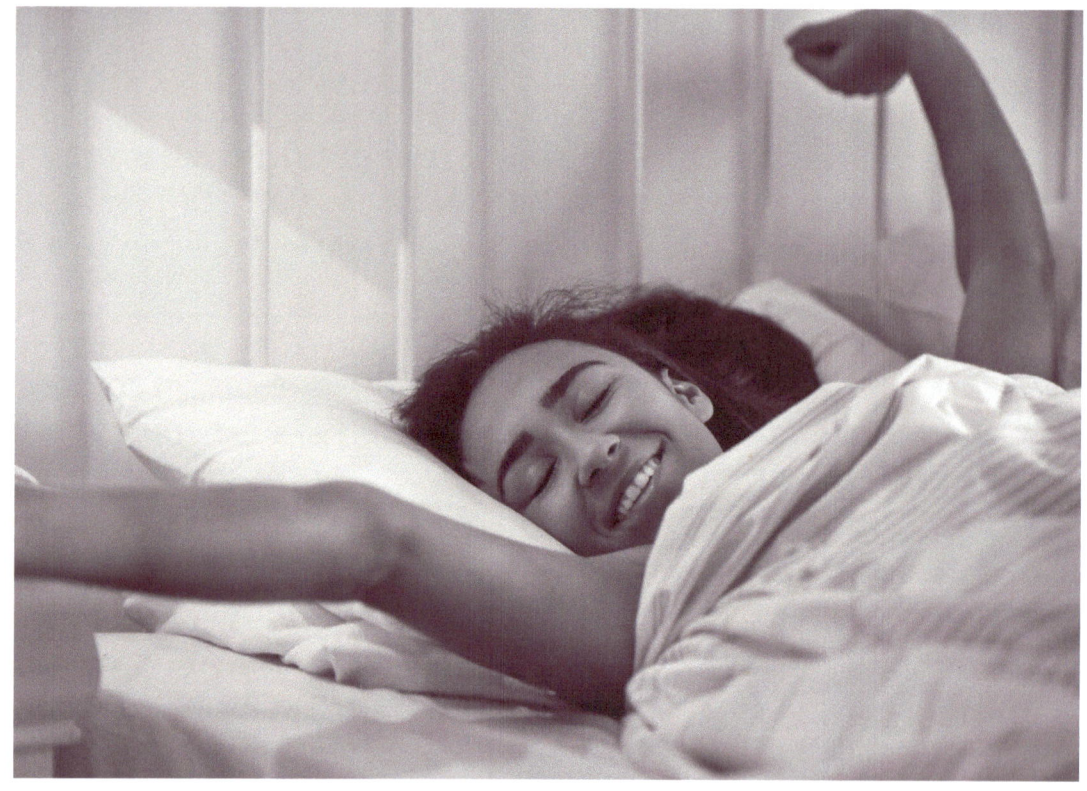

Acknowledging your child's great feelings from sleep, empowers them to embrace their Sleep Wellness superpowers.

15: Allow your child to sleep until they awake naturally.

> **PARENT HACK:**
> If tweens or teens sleep in late on weekends, holidays, or vacations, they are not being lazy. They are making up their sleep debt, which is a good thing. *They cannot sleep so much if no sleep debt is owed.*

This advice might make you wish your parents had taken this approach with you, especially when you were a tween or teenager on the weekends!

Can you recall a time as a child when all you wanted to do was catch up on your sleep and were labeled lazy? As an adult, can you not sleep as long as you want because you hear that voice calling you lazy?

Well, allowing children to sleep until they are ready to greet the world on their own helps ensure they have slept to their full quota, which is required for healthy growth and repair.

If lingering in bed past the time for school is commonplace, for example, it is best to make bedtime earlier to accommodate the extra sleep they need. A disciplined plan of sleeping earlier in the evening is a strategically sound and efficient approach to making up for lost sleep or repaying their sleep debt accumulated over time.

A healthy person who has slept enough and awakened refreshed over several days cannot sleep during the day—even if you paid them. So, if you are concerned your child is sleeping more than usual, this need for sleep is driven by sleep debt, illness, or a growth spurt.

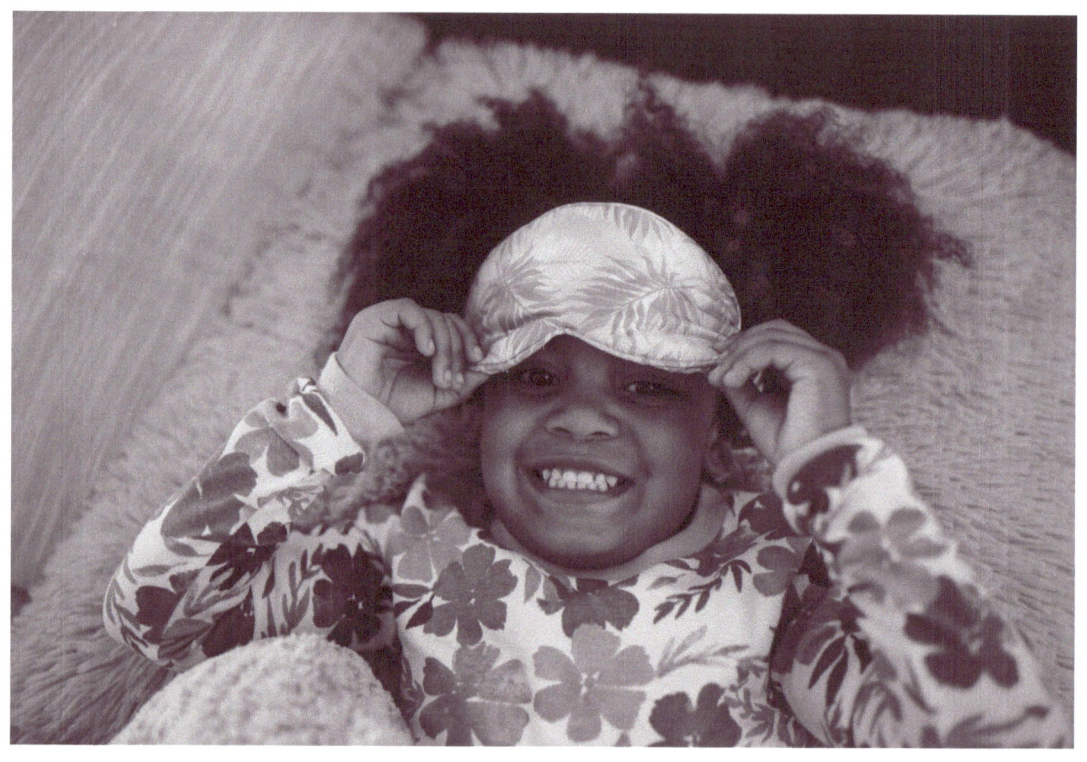

The most critical, good habit of Sleep Wellness is doing everything possible to provide a safe space for your child to sleep at the appropriate time with minimal disturbance and free from concern.

16: Celebrate when your child feels great after sleeping well and feeling refreshed.

> **PARENT HACK:**
> Deepening your child's relationship with sleep in this way entrains them to appreciate and hold dear their ability to sleep well and model their superpower of Sleep Wellness for the rest of the family.

Acknowledging your child's good feelings from sleep empowers them to embrace their Sleep Wellness *superpowers*.

Together, when you observe and treasure how magical sleep can be after their illness, a tough day at school, or just being tired from playing, it enables them to associate sleep with a natural source of energy and power—which they naturally have access to.

17: Provide a safe space to make the most of the wonders and magic of sleep.

> **PARENT HACK:**
> Observe your young child and engage in conversations as they grow older to confirm their sense of safety in their sleeping environment.

All living beings on Earth seek a **safe place** for their offspring to sleep peacefully and grow, finding comfort amidst life's challenges. While human parents naturally prioritize this need with infants, they may relax their guard as children grow older. It's crucial to trust your instincts and remain watchful.

Ensuring that your child feels secure and at ease when going to bed, regardless of the hardships faced by adults in the household, eases their worries.

Providing a secure haven where your child can seek solace and tap into the wonder and magic of sleep helps them strengthen themselves and develop resilience.

Regardless of how 'wealthy' or 'poor' your circumstances are, strive to enhance your child's comfort and maintain their safety during sleep. Encourage them to confide in you if their sleeping space no longer feels safe and secure.

Part 5

SET A GOOD EXAMPLE: SUPPORT FOR ADULTS IN THE HOUSEHOLD

18: Kickstarting Sleep Wellness begins with you. (Page 42-43)

19: Yes, you can set standards for your children. (Page 44)

20: Children need you to hold the line. (Page 45)

21: We are sounding the alarm for night owls. (Page 46-47)

22: Sleep debt is your silent threat. (Page 48)

23: Pay your sleep debt. (Page 49)

24: Sleep-debt free reaps enormous dividends. (Page 50)

25: When time runs short, it is fool's gold to stay up late. (Page 51)

26: Forego the night and make early mornings a family affair! (Page 52-54)

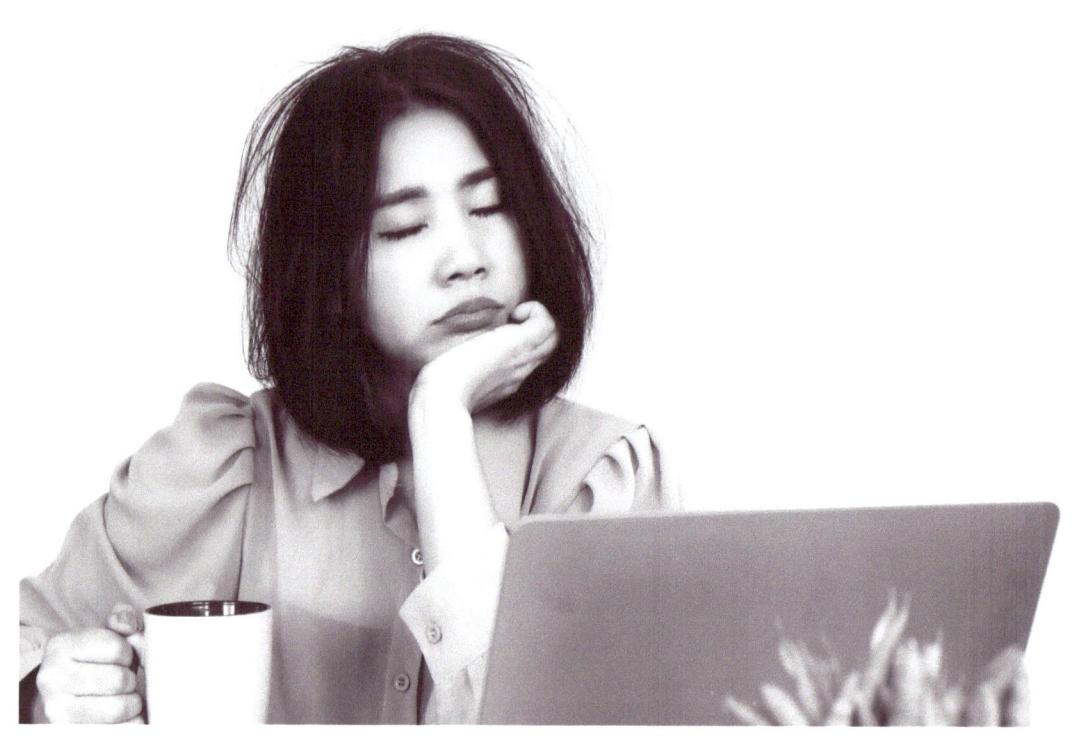

Most adults downgrade sleep to the point of ignoring it. They put it off until it overtakes them, making it harder to break bad habits and adopt good Sleep Wellness ones.

18: Kickstarting Sleep Wellness begins with you.

Most adults are victims of sleep trauma.

Let's begin with some grace. Adults today face enormous pressure from generational sleep trauma, cultural myths, and personal habits that undermine sleep.

We've inherited cultural messages that glorify productivity and dismiss sleep as a sign of laziness.

Many of us have internalized the belief that staying up late to finish chores—or indulge in well-earned "me time"—is both necessary and normal, even virtuous. But over time, this pattern erodes our body's natural ability to fall asleep easily and stay asleep deeply.

By age 20, the average adult loses 10 minutes of sleep per decade. By age 60, sleep time plateaus at just 6.5–7 hours per night.

This is in stark contrast to centenarians in Blue Zones—like Loma Linda—who sleep 7 to 8+ hours nightly, often supplemented by restorative daytime naps. They live longer and healthier in part because they sleep more.

However, it is never too late, and no improvement in Sleep Wellness is too small to make a difference in your children's overall health and well-being, or in yours.

19: Yes, you can set standards for your children.

We often expect children to follow rules we ourselves don't follow. That's not hypocrisy—it's parenting. Just as children are restricted from adult behaviors like alcohol and tobacco, they also deserve protection from the cultural sleep sabotage many of us have normalized.

The truth is, most parents want more for their children than they managed for themselves. Sleep should be no exception.

> *"My experience as a physician is that people will often do for their families what they cannot do for themselves."*

That includes safeguarding their child's sleep—even while their own suffers. You may not be able to model perfect sleep habits, but you can protect your child from absorbing a culture that devalues sleep. That's a powerful gift.

For most modern adults, Sleep Wellness feels impractical. But for children, it's foundational.

20: Children need you to hold the line.

While it's true that children are more likely to mirror what they see, it's also true that standards help children thrive—especially when it comes to sleep.

Letting kids "get away" with staying up late may feel harmless at first. But once they associate being awake past their sleep window with freedom, pleasure, or reward, they begin to crave it. It becomes a reinforced behavior, difficult to undo.

When bedtime becomes negotiable, Sleep Wellness becomes optional—and that's a problem. Staying up late disrupts the circadian rhythm and shortens the time spent in the deepest, most restorative stages of sleep. It chips away at the very systems that support emotional regulation, immune function, memory, and physical growth.

Holding a firm sleep boundary—even when it's not mirrored—is part of your essential caregiving. It's how you protect the possibility of lifelong sleep wellness for your child.

> **FAMILY SLEEP WELLNESS HACK:**
> For your children's sake, maintain a standard of prioritizing Sleep Wellness as strictly as you can, for as long as you can.

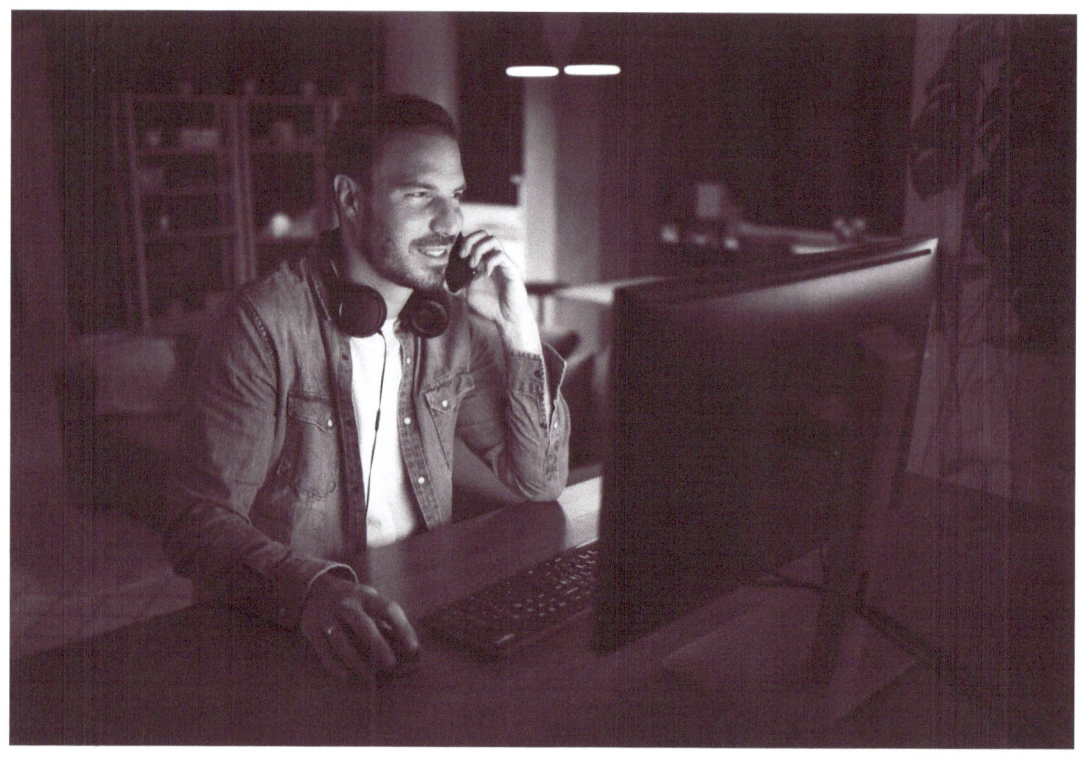

If you are a night owl, you stay up late to get your me-time. <u>This type of me-time isn't self-care.</u> It's the opposite. Ignoring your sleep cues today means you're less productive tomorrow.

21: We are sounding the alarm for night owls.

"TRANKY": The hidden cost of Night Owl habits.

Late-night scrolling or chores may feel like freedom, but it quietly drains your reserves. What seems like *"me time"* can leave you tired, reactive, and emotionally off the next day—a state I call:

TRANKY (tired, trippin', and cranky)

Sleep-deprived adults often misread situations, feel overwhelmed, and struggle to stay present—even when trying their best. It's a cycle of late-night reward and next-day regret that affects not just you, but everyone around you.

It's no wonder that sleep-deprived adults often crave the jolt of energy and fleeting excitement that comes from pushing past the natural sleep window, the 'Washington Sleep Wellness Window', and indulging in late-night distractions. But come morning, they are met with the weight of not feeling like 'a morning person.'

It's a cycle many of us know too well. Recognizing this pattern is the first step toward restoring sleep, presence, and a more stable emotional landscape—for your family and you.

22: Sleep debt is the silent threat.

Do you know how much Sleep Debt you have?

Many physical, emotional, and cognitive complaints are signs of one common problem: sleep debt. Sufficient sleep is foundational to wellness, and without enough of it, your body's systems begin to misfire—even if you don't immediately notice.

If you:

- **Wake up groggy or tired.**
- **Feel like you're moving through the day in a fog.**
- **Get sleepy after lunch or need a nap to keep going.**
- **Feel unusually irritable, impatient, or emotionally reactive.**
- **Feel less motivated or capable than usual.**
- **Wake up achy or gaining weight without explanation.**
- **Feel anxious, unmotivated, or feel depressive for no reason.**
- **Find yourself catching colds or getting sick more often.**
- **Feeling your best in the late evening or at night.**

Then you most likely have sleep debt.

The good news? You can reverse it!

Prioritize your sleep in accordance with your circadian rhythm. It is the most efficient way to restore your system.

Sleep debt doesn't have to become a permanent deficit.

23: Pay your sleep debt

It is simple: Get more sleep to pay back sleep debt.

Sleep debt is real—and most of us carry it. But here's the good news: even a few extra hours of sleep on a weekend, or during a break in your schedule, can help restore balance and relieve the physiological and emotional toll of chronic under-sleeping.

> **SLEEP HACK:**
> Resolve to sleep as early as you can, for as long as you can whenever you can.

Some people wake from extra sleep and feel guilty, thinking they've been lazy. If after sleeping longer, you still feel groggy, it's absolutely because you still have sleep debt.

It's a myth that you can sleep too long or that it could be harmful.

Extra sleep is for repair and growth—same as in children, maturing teens, and people recovering from illness. Think about what you have been missing..

24: Sleep-debt free reaps enormous dividends.

Around the world, long-lived communities known as Blue Zones enjoy not only longer lifespans but also greater day-to-day wellness. One overlooked factor? Their cultural alignment with circadian rhythms and their reverence for the evening wind-down.

In these cultures, evenings are not for entertainment, but for relaxing and restoring. Instead of chasing stimulation, people pursue inner calm—sharing food, enjoying their family, and their community. They honor a period of self-reflection and gratitude. This rhythm protects sleep and encourages deep connection—both within families and within oneself.

The effects are enormous: lower rates of illness, greater emotional resilience, and an enduring sense of purpose. As you feel the effects of renewed energy from deeper, more consistent sleep, something powerful happens—your urge to distract yourself with entertainment becomes weaker, and your relationship with sleep and its benefits grows stronger.

When you prioritize sleep, you're not just resting your muscles—you're choosing health, energy, and longevity. The dividends are not just physical. They're spiritual and emotional. And they compound across generations.

25: When time runs short, it's fool's gold to stay up late.

> **PARENT HACK:**
> If you only have time to sleep 5–6 hours, listen to your body's cues, go to sleep in alignment with your circadian rhythm, and cheat the morning sleep—not the night.

Adults in the family often feel there simply aren't enough hours to get everything done, let alone sleep eight hours!

However, pushing through your fatigue to stay up late costs you far more than it returns!

That "second wind" you feel at 10 or 11 p.m.? It's a trap. It brings alertness at the exact moment your body should be preparing for its deepest and most healing sleep.

If you override that window when it opens, you miss the rich, early-night deep sleep your body needs to repair, regulate mood, and replenish energy. Instead, you experience a lighter, more fragmented phase of sleep—less restful, less restorative, which triggers illness and disease.

Know your cues. You're better off going to bed when your body first says it's ready.

Yawning, eye rubbing, eyelid heaviness, a wave of stillness—those are signs your Washington Sleep Wellness Window is open. Embrace it, and resolve to tackle your tasks feeling clearer, calmer, and more capable in the morning.

As a bonus, you'll often accomplish more the next day with less effort than you would by staying up chasing productivity at night.

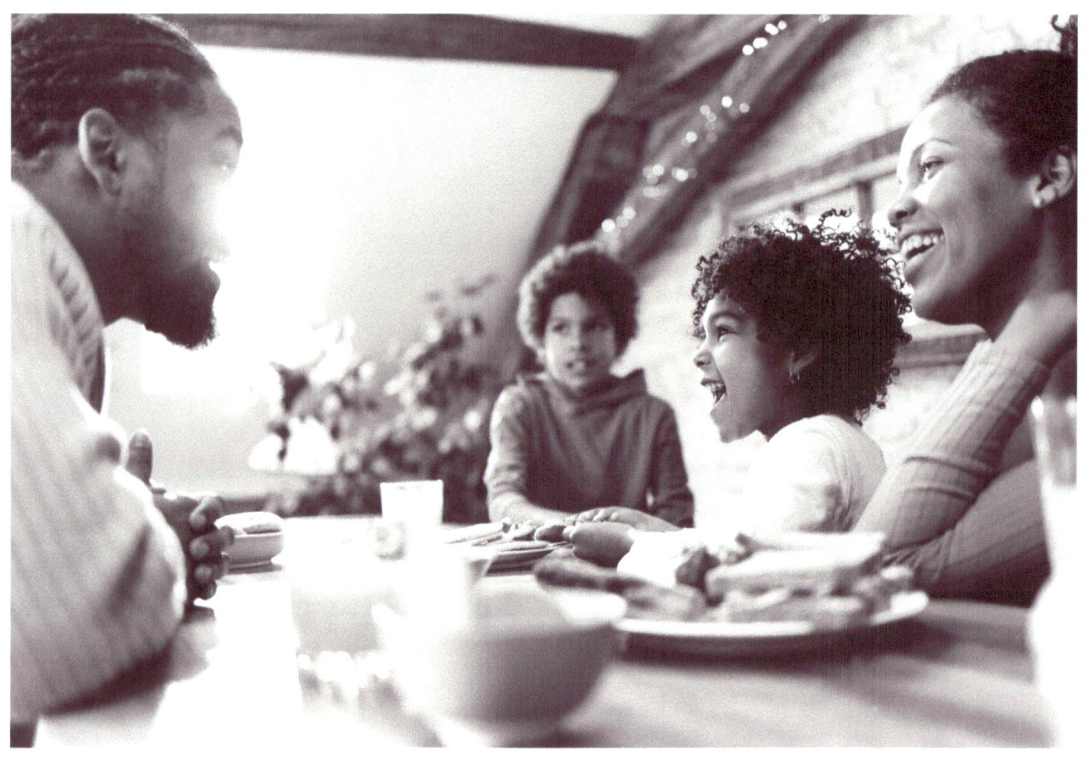

When you stop being a night owl, you can enjoy higher quality time connecting in the morning over breakfast and even doing chores or homework instead of staying up late and soldiering on.

26: Forego the night and make early mornings a family affair!

> **PARENT HACK:**
> Quality time spent with your family after great sleep is both priceless and memorable!

As you plan to have more time in the morning when you are fresher, think more clearly, and are more capable and efficient, chores and homework can be done with less drudgery.

If that movie, news, or sporting event is so important, record it so you can watch it in the morning.

Most parents who start to covet deep sleep earlier at night find they are less frivolous with their time in the morning. They also find that the shows they used to stay up late to watch were less funny and exciting, and sports they felt they could not miss before bed were less important than spending higher quality time with their family.

As your children mature and have more evening activities, meals and gatherings become less consistent.

Everyone is likelier to be together in the morning, whatever your circumstances.

If your morning family routine is usually a rushed blur, it does not have to be when you awake refreshed and energized.

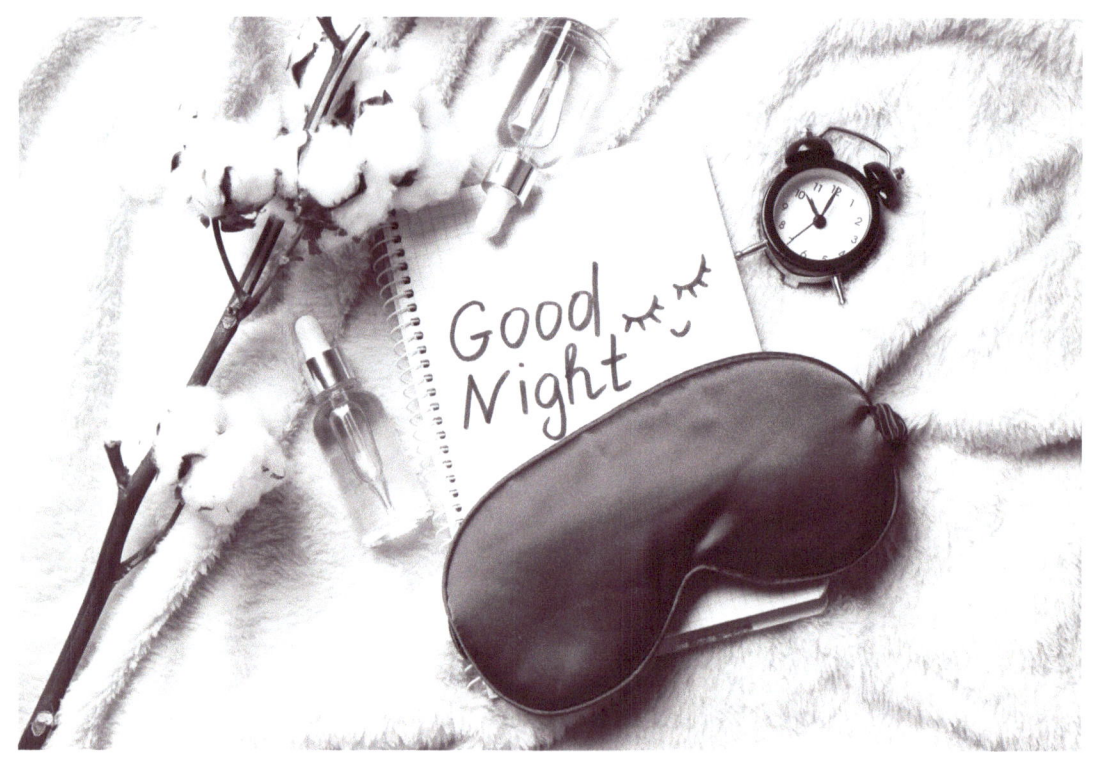

Parents, you know the basics to feeling better. It is the same as if you were recovering from any illness: Exercise appropriately, drink enough water, say no to alcohol and junk food, eat better, and <u>GET GREAT SLEEP!</u>

More Good Sleep Wellness Stuff

Frequently Asked Questions (Page 56-58)

Glossary (Page 59-60)

Recommended Additional Reading (Page 61)

Get our 'Kid-Approved' Bedtime Storybook (Page 62)

Help Sound the Alarm for Sleep Wellness (Page 63)

Contact Us (Page 64)

Frequently Asked Questions

What about parents who work the second and third shifts, coming home after bedtime and disturbing the children?

Consider resisting the urge to unwind, catching your *second wind*, and indulging in *me-time*. Prioritize your children's best interest – and yours – and try to come in quietly and prepare for bed right away. If you are quiet but still disturb the children, don't worry, it will only be momentary. They will go back to sleep when you are also settled in. If the children are in another room away from light, limit the noise of late-night TV watching with headphones. However, immediately going to bed increases the chances that you can wake up and enjoy the morning with the children.

How do I put to bed my youngest child who shares a room with the older ones who go to bed two hours later?

This is much more challenging after the younger one has gotten a taste of staying up past bedtime to hang out with the older siblings. If this is the case, the rule-setting is best rolled out with a new ritual that makes the younger one feel special, like reading a book, a coloring activity, bathtime, etc., because they are special! Sleep is doing very special things to their bodies, minds, emotions, dreams, aspirations, and imaginations. As a parent, you don't want them to miss out! Once in bed, the younger ones can don their own special eye mask and headphones. The older child needs to take responsibility and tone down their activity to respect the younger one's sleep needs and use headphones for the electronics, which they may be eager to do as a role model.

Frequently Asked Questions

After all the kids are in bed, nighttime is my only time to get things done. Even when I'm tired, I catch a second wind. Isn't that my body telling me I have the energy?

Yes, you have the energy, but you are borrowing the energy and running a sleep debt you must repay at some point. Repayment can come from withholding energy to support your immune system, energy to heal when you fall sick, the energy you need to problem-solve, and the energy you need to be resilient mentally and emotionally. We are all energy borrowers in our modern world, especially in the United States! I advise paying your sleep debt by making time to catch up on your sleep and sleeping in without any alarms for as long as you need. Limit your energy borrowing by going to bed earlier and waking up earlier for me-time.

If sleep is so important, why hasn't my doctor asked me about my child's sleep during exams?

Traditional medical schools train doctors to treat illnesses when symptoms appear, not preventive medicine. Sufficient sleep keeps you healthier; when you are not getting it, many symptoms of illness can arise. Through my Foundation, I am providing Sleep Wellness tools for doctors to proactively engage parents about their children's sleep habits and draw the connection between their illnesses and lack of sufficient sleep. Our tools are based on using sufficient sleep to treat various illnesses and diseases in my medical practice.

Frequently Asked Questions

How long will it take for my family to see results from our new Sleep Wellness habits?

You will likely see immediate results in your children's behaviors. They will feel more energetic, upbeat, and eager to start their day the more they adopt the habit of honoring their bedtime and sleeping when they are first drowsy and undisturbed for as long as possible.

It may take longer for the adults in the household to feel the euphoria of Sleep Wellness because busy adults who resist sleep carry more sleep debt than children and may take longer to repay sleep debt. However, there is no doubt that every bit of extra sleep you get will make a difference, and it is never too late to catch up on your sleep.

Even changing your attitude toward sleep can go a long way to restore you. Chip away at your sleep debt by intending to welcome sleep when you feel drowsy, being passionate about waking up refreshed, going to bed when you recognize your sleep cues, or taking a morning to sleep as late as possible.

As an adult, you may find it more challenging to break sabotaging habits ingrained during childhood and later by society as a working adult. However, so many of my patients find it easier to reap the reward of Sleep Wellness with each small step they take.

Glossary

Lack of Sufficient Sleep
Lack of Sufficient Sleep, LOSS, is the root cause of disease. LOSS weakens the immune system, opening the door to minor and major infections and cancers. LOSS triggers metabolic changes that result in metabolic illnesses. LOSS also triggers autoimmune diseases. Sufficient sleep strengthens the immune system, acting as a preventive medicine and a healing agent to restore health. Sufficient sleep strengthens and restores every aspect of the body and mind, promoting longevity, good health, and a feeling of physical and mental well-being.

Night Owls
I call them *'Energy Borrowers'*—people who get extra energy and feel productive in the late evening and midnight hours. They usually describe themselves as "not a morning person." If the debt goes unpaid, they become more susceptible to mistakes made while fatigued, the drudgery of feeling tired so often, depressive thought processes, and eventually metabolic and inflammatory illnesses.

Second Wind
The *second wind* describes the increase in energy you experience when fighting off the urge to sleep in the evening. With the increase in energy comes a pleasant feeling of giddiness and less drowsiness. (My Persian patients have shared an apt phrase in Farsi, *hobbish paridewind burst of energy, and it feels exciting, like a treat,* which means "sleepiness jumps up and flies away.") If your child stays up past their natural sleep window, they are likely to get a second, and that rush creates an addictive craving. When bedtime becomes negotiable, kids start to chase that feeling. Staying consistent helps children and adults fall asleep more easily and keeps natural rhythms on track.

Glossary

Sleep Cues
There are physical, mental, and emotional signals that you need to sleep. These natural signs often go unnoticed: yawning, eye rubbing, nodding, head bobbing, head scratching, drowsiness, crankiness, and irritability.

Sleep Debt
If you feel sleepy and can sleep, your body needs it. A person can sleep up to what their sleep debt demands. In other words, once you pay back your sleep debt, you will awake and be unable to sleep more. Dr. William Dement, a Stanford professor often called the father of the sleep hygiene movement, refuted the commonly held notion that people may sleep because they are bored. In one of Dr. Dement's studies, where students were required to lay in bed in the dark 12 hours per day for two weeks, he noticed many students initially slept 12 hours. Still, by the 11th day, all the students slept no more than eight hours because their sleep debt was paid. In my practice, I observed that patients who accumulated sleep debt were most likely to increase their chance of illness.

Tranky
The combination of 'tired' and 'cranky' that results from LOSS.

Washington Sleep Wellness Window
The 'window of opportunity' for a great night's sleep opens when your sleep cues appear and closes shut (and is difficult to reopen) after the second wind kicks in.

Recommended Additional Reading

Franco, P. et al (Seret, N., Van Hees, J., Scaillet, S., Vermeulen, F., Grosswasser, J., Jahn, A.) **Decreased Arousals in Healthy Infants After Short-term Sleep Deprivation Pediatrics** 2004 Aug;114(2):e192-7

Washington, Roger W., MD with Nickhol, Scarlet B., MPP, MBA (2015). **Lack of Sufficient Sleep Matters: Decode the Root Cause of Your Illness,** CreateSpace Independent Publishing, Silicon Valley, CA.

Entrain Your Child to Sleep Wellness
Our Bedtime Storybook

Instilling an appreciation for sleep in young children will serve them throughout their lives. It is a gift that will keep on giving. In his family practice, Dr. Washington observed how difficult it was for older children and adults to break bad habits, but young children were more eager to learn and adapt. Children and their caregivers, especially those touched by adverse childhood experiences, are the primary concern of the Sleep To Live Well Foundation educational materials, one of which is our delightful children's book:

Help children eagerly embrace Sleep Wellness habits.

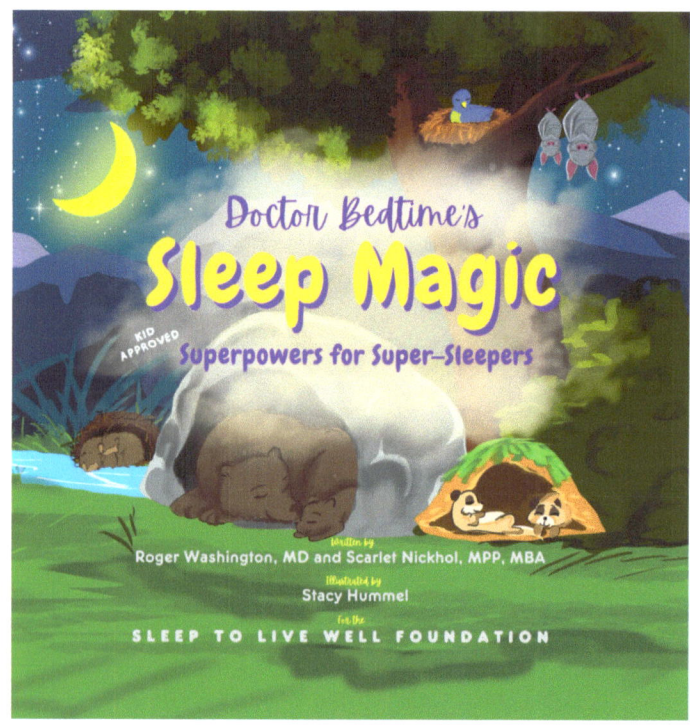

Front Cover

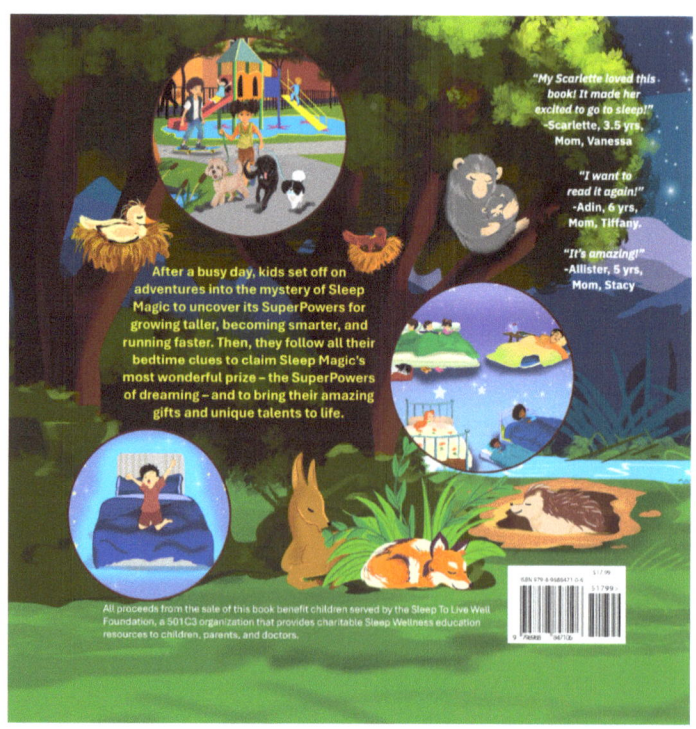

Back Cover

This bedtime story is designed for reading to children between 2 and 9. It is brimming with enchanting rhymes, couplets, and beautiful illustrations that capture their imagination. The book follows the sleep journey of a diverse and multicultural cast of characters and is 38 pages long. Throughout the story, children will learn about sleep's *wonders and magic,* including how it helps them grow, heal, energize, and learn. It teaches life lessons about **listening to your body** for sleep cues and **having a safe space** to drift away, both cornerstones of Sleep Wellness.

By answering W*here,* W*hy,* and W*hen* we sleep, Dr. Roger Washington, aka Doctor Bedtime, deepens a child's relationship with sleep as a source of empowerment for physical, mental, and emotional well-being. Whimsically told, this colorful story is a wonderful way to make children eager to keep their appointments with bedtime!

Find out more at our website: www.SleepToLiveWell.org

Proceeds from this book and the Parents Sleep Wellness Guide, which the non-profit organization Sleep To Live Well Foundation publishes, and all other donations go toward expanding our charitable programs.

Help Sound the Alarm for Sleep Wellness

GET INVOLVED!

Help sound the alarm for Sleep Wellness.

Visit our website at **www.SleepToLiveWell.org** and learn how we are **sounding the alarm** about insufficient sleep as the root cause of illness. We also offer the guidance and education that children, parents, and physicians need to embrace Sleep Wellness for a healthier world.

Support our charitable programs to help children build resiliency and make the lemonade out of lemons they may encounter in life.

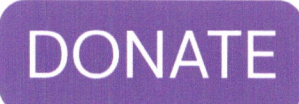

Contact Us

We would love to hear how our Parents Guide supports your Sleep Wellness journey.

Email:
info@sleeptolivewell.org

Write:
2365 Quimby Rd Ste 260
San Jose, CA 95122

Call:
1.888.395.7794

Executive Director
Chief Marketing Officer
Scarlet B Nickhol, MPP, MBA

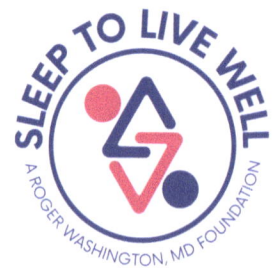

WWW.SLEEPTOLIVEWELL.ORG

www.ingramcontent.com/pod-product-compliance
Lightning Source LLC
Chambersburg PA
CBHW061156030426
42337CB00002B/20